I0428998

BREATHING :

TECHNIQUES FOR HAPPINESS AND HEALTHY LIVING

By Rita Singh

Copyright © 2016

© Copyright 2016 by The Canberra Writing Group - All rights reserved.

This document is geared towards providing exact and reliable information in regards to the topic and issue covered. The publication is sold with the idea that the publisher is not required to render accounting, officially permitted, or otherwise, qualified services. If advice is necessary, legal or professional, a practiced individual in the profession should be ordered.

- From a Declaration of Principles which was accepted and approved equally by a Committee of the American Bar Association and a Committee of Publishers and Associations.

In no way is it legal to reproduce, duplicate, or transmit any part of this document in either electronic means or in printed format. Recording of this publication is strictly prohibited and any storage of this document is not allowed unless with written permission from the publisher. All rights reserved.

The information provided herein is stated to be truthful and consistent, in that any liability, in terms of inattention or otherwise, by any usage or abuse of any policies, processes, or directions contained within is the solitary and utter responsibility of the recipient reader. Under no circumstances will any legal responsibility or blame be held against the publisher for any reparation, damages, or monetary loss due to the information herein, either directly or indirectly.

Respective authors own all copyrights not held by the publisher.

The information herein is offered for informational purposes solely, and is universal as so. The presentation of the information is without contract or any type of guarantee assurance.

The trademarks that are used are without any consent, and the publication of the trademark is without permission or backing by the trademark owner. All trademarks and brands within this book are for clarifying purposes only and are the owned by the owners themselves, not affiliated with this document.

Introduction

In order to understand why proper breathing is so vital to maintaining a healthy life, it is helpful to understand that the body is a complex biological machine. Any machine you can think of, whether mechanical or genetic, needs energy to run. In addition, it needs the proper kind of energy, delivered in a specific way, in order to run efficiently. A car, for example, is designed to mix a certain amount of gas with oxygen in order for it to run effectively.

When a spark is added a controlled explosion occurs which generates energy. It is this energy that turns the drive shaft and propels the car forward. What happens though, if the car is fed low quality fuel or if the oxygen and gas are mixed in less than their ideal proportions? You guessed it: the car will not perform well or may not even run at all.

When it comes to generating energy our bodies are not that different from cars. Our bodies produce energy by combining fuel (carbohydrates) and oxygen in appropriate proportions. This mixture is then burned, similar to a car, in order to produce life energy. The only real difference between the two is that your body burns its fuel at a much slower and lower temperature. What is important to remember though is, just like a car, if your body is fed poor food or air quality, or if it is not mixed correctly, your body will run poorly as well. Whereas your car will stall, you as a biological machine will likely feel drowsy and fatigued. What's even worse is that as you are burning your fuel inefficiently you will likely wind up storing more of it in the form of fat.

The second way that deep breathing promotes health is through the elimination of toxins from the body. It does this by expelling carbon dioxide and other waste products when you exhale, which most people understand. What most people don't understand however is that proper breathing is also critical to a properly functioning lymphatic system.

Your body contains lymph fluid, which is used to purge waste and debris from your system. Under some circumstances if your lymphatic system shuts down for whatever reason, you would literally poison yourself within 24 hours and die. What is different about your lymphatic system is that it has no pump to circulate fluid throughout the body. It is completely reliant on body movement and breathing to circulate. By helping to keep your lymphatic system working at peak efficiency breathing remains to be one of the most important things we can do as human beings.

Table of Contents

CHAPTER 1: HAPPINESS, BREATHING AND THE MIND

Only a small percentage of people truly understand the relationship between proper breathing and health (both physically and mentally). The truth is that your breath is the road that connects your mind with body. Consider this: When you are calm and relaxed so is your breathing. On the other hand when you are stressed or panicking your breathing typically becomes more frequent and shallow.

I've seen some yogi's, who are experts at breath control, seemingly be able to read minds by simply observing the person's breath. What is interesting though is that the mind body connection is a two way street. If you are not aware of it your "monkey mind" tends to control your breathing.

However, when you are aware of this fact you can actually use your breath to calm your mind. Mental states involving stress, insomnia, anxiety, panic attacks and depression can all be greatly mitigated if not eliminated by learning to calm your mind by controlling your breath. Calm, slow deep breathing is the key.

CHAPTER 2: HOW DO YOU BREATHE PROPERLY?

In order to understand why there are so many benefits to breathing properly we need to look at the process of breathing itself. The first thing to know is that the nose is designed to be the primary system by which we inhale and exhale our breath, unlike our mouth. It is designed to clean and prepare the air before it reaches our lungs. Here's how it does this. When air first enters the nose it must first pass through nasal hair, which helps to filter out any fine particles.

The air then passes over three seashell like structures called turbinates. The turbinates job is to stir up the incoming air and force it to circulate over a much larger surface than would otherwise be the case. This helps to correct the air temperature (either heating it up or cooling it down) and humidity level so that it is ideally suited to enter the delicate lungs. In addition to this, the interior of the nose is also coated with a constantly moving mucous membrane that is able to absorb dust, bacteria and viruses.

Most people are only aware of this membrane when they are sick and might experience a runny nose and phlegm buildup. What inevitably happens is that some mucous is prone to move to the back of the throat. Once there, it can be swallowed into the stomach where any sort of bacteria and/or viruses are destroyed. The air then leaves the nose (or mouth) and enters the trachea, otherwise known as the windpipe. The trachea then splits in two, one for each lung. Like branches on a tree, the bronchi continue to split, getting smaller and smaller. After about 15 generations, the bronchi shrink into microscopic bronchioles, which are attached to very tiny air sacs called alveoli.

These air sacs are so small that the lung tissue only appears to be solid to the naked eye. In reality, they are only a single cell thick and very membranous. It is here where the oxygen exchange takes place with the tiny blood vessels known as capillaries. In fact the capillaries are so small that individual blood cells have to squeeze through them in a single file manner. Now how do we use this knowledge in order to maximize your bodies' energy production? The key thing to remember is that your lungs are shaped similarly to a triangle, with a large base becoming narrower as it reaches the top. In order to maximize the oxygen exchange and therefore your body's energy production you want to ensure that it is the base of your lungs that are constantly being filled with fresh oxygen. As the base of your lungs contain the widest surface area, this ensures that the maximum oxygen exchange takes place.

Now that we understand the importance of maximizing the oxygen exchange process we need to look at the three different types of breathing you can perform and how we can use this to our benefit. The first type of breathing is known as diaphragmatic breathing. The diaphragm is the large muscle located below the lungs that separates the thorax from the abdomen. When it is relaxed this muscle bulges upward in a dome shape which compresses the lungs. When we contract the diaphragm it becomes a flat disc. This expands the lungs from the bottom and allows for the greatest amount of air to enter.

The second type of breathing you can perform is known as chest breathing. This involves the intercostal muscles, which are the muscles that are attached to the ribs. When they are activated, the rib cage expands allowing air into the upper and middle sections of the lungs. The third type of breathing is known as clavicle breathing. This involves pulling the clavicles (collarbone) muscles upwards. It is used to get air into the very top of the lungs. From what you know now it should be noted that of these three breathing methods, you should challenge yourself to engage in diaphragmatic breathing as frequently as possible.

Chest and clavicle breathing should only be used when the body is under severe stress, for example, after participating in strenuous sports. Even then, chest and clavicle breathing should only be used in conjunction with diaphragmatic breathing, not replacing it.

Let's get started!

We are now ready to begin exploring various kinds of deep breathing exercises. Before we do though, I want to stress the importance of not taking these exercises lightly. Before you begin any exercise program, including this one, I highly recommend that you talk to your doctor first. This is especially true if you have any form of high blood pressure. As you read through these exercises you will see that many of them involve holding your breath for short periods of time.

If you do have high blood pressure, I would recommend that you NOT begin holding your breath until you discuss it with your doctor. The act of holding your breath will cause your blood pressure to rise. If this is an issue for you, you will need to approach it with extreme caution. Another general rule you should take into account: never force any of these exercises. If you are feeling faint or dizzy at anytime simply stop and take a break until the feeling passes. It may take your body some time to get used to breathing properly. So it is important that you don't rush the process and allow a natural and organic progression to practicing these techniques.

CHAPTER 3: BASIC DIAPHRAGMATIC BREATHING

Now that you know why proper deep breathing is so important for your health and mental wellbeing, we can now start training your body to be able to perform it properly. What follows is a lesson on how to do basic diaphragmatic breathing along with some variations involving various hand positions and nasal breathing exercises. Always remember that proper diaphragmatic breathing is not meant to be done only at specific times. Rather, you should try to make it good habit to breathe from your diaphragm with deep slow breaths throughout the day. If you are ever feeling stressed, take a moment and analyze how you are breathing. We tend to neglect thinking about our breathing patterns because we're so caught up in daily life. By focusing on your breath you will begin to feel better in no time.

CHAPTER 4: HOW TO PERFORM A DIAPHRAGMATIC BREATH

Before you attempt your first proper diaphragmatic breath you will want to assume a comfortable deep breathing posture which can mean standing, sitting, or lying flat on the floor. If you are standing or seated try rocking slightly from side to side in order to align your tailbone with the top of your head. You should feel as if the weight of your head is directly above your spinal column. To accomplish this you may need to pull your chin up slightly.

Remember that with whatever posture you assume, you want your back to be comfortably straight but not rigid.

Once you are relaxed perform the following:

1. Begin to breathe exclusively through your nose by placing your tongue on the roof of your mouth while keeping your mouth closed.

2. Place your left hand on your chest and your right hand on your abdomen just be- low your belly button.

3. Begin to inhale through your nose for a count of 5. As you do so, visualize your diaphragm pulling down and expanding. At the same time use your minds eye to imagine clean, pure air flowing into your nose and filling your lungs. Keep other thoughts and

distractions out the picture. Simply focus on your breathing

4. Hold this breath for a count of 7.

5. Exhale through your nose for a count of 8 and repeat.

As you exhale imagine that you are expelling toxic gas in some form. As you inhale and exhale pay attention to your hands. If you are performing this deep diaphragmatic breath correctly the hand on your abdomen should always be the first to move, not the one on your chest. Your aim is to always have your lungs fill up with oxygen from the bottom up, never the top down. Visualizing your breath in some form is very important as well. The incoming breath is the energizing breath; while the outgoing breath will help you relieve tension and stress.

CHAPTER 5: HAND POSTURES FOR DEEPER MEDITATION

Once you are confident that you are performing the deep diaphragmatic breath correctly you will want to incorporate some of these hand positions to enhance your practice. In India these are called *Mudras* and they can have a subtle yet powerful affect on the mind/body connection.

Prayer Seal (Anjali Mudra)

To perform this mudra gently put your two palms together with your thumbs placed against your breastbone. By joining your hands together in this manner you are making a physical gesture that you recognize the interconnectedness of all living things. This mudra is thought to be calming as it helps to harmonize the left and right hemispheres of the brain.

Chin Mudra

To perform this mudra you will want to touch your thumb to your index finger with your palms facing downwards. In many yoga texts the index finger represents the soul and the thumb represents universal consciousness. By bringing your fingers together in this manner, it is said that you are allowing your soul to get in touch with a higher power. Having your palm face down helps to seal in the awareness of this higher consciousness.

Gyana Mudra

This mudra is similar to the Chin Mudra with the exception that it is performed with the palms facing upward. In yoga texts this helps to calm the mind while sealing in wisdom.

Hakini Mudra

This mudra is said to help with thinking and concentration by aiding in the coordination between the right and left centers of the brain. It can be practiced anywhere at any time. It is particularly useful when you need to clear your mind. If you are having difficulty recalling a fact or thought, practicing the Hakini Mudra can often help you remember it. To perform the Hakini Mudra do the following:

1. Hold your hands in front of you with your palms facing each other. Do not bring your palms together, however.

2. Touch the fingertips of your right hand with their counterparts on your left.

3. When you perform your diaphragmatic breath, inhale through your nose with your tongue against the roof of your mouth.

4. When you exhale through your nose allow your tongue to relax.

Yoni Mudra

With this mudra you will be creating a downward facing triangle with your hands, which is meant to symbolize the womb as a source of life energy. This mudra will calm your mind and will allow you to relax as you focus on your breath work.

1. Begin with your hands resting just below your navel.
2. Interlock your fingers and spread your hands slightly.
3. Straighten your index fingers so that they are pointed downwards with the tips touching.

4. Touch the tips of your thumbs together and straighten them as well.

CHAPTER 6: RELAXATION TECHNIQUES – NASAL BREATHING

The final basic diaphragmatic breathing variation we will look at involves alternate nostril breathing. You are likely not aware of this but your body is constantly rotating between nostrils when you breathe. This allows one nostril to recharge while the opposite is performing the primary function of purifying the incoming air.

To yogis and many other deep breathing practitioners this alternating nostril-breathing pattern actually affects your mind as well. Through thousands of years of practice they have come to believe that the left nostril accesses the right hemisphere of the brain. This is the feminine, cooling side of the brain that is most often associated with creative and dreamy thoughts. Your right nostril is associated with your left, masculine side of your brain.

This part of the brain is the analytical, competitive side of your mind. By consciously alternating your nasal breathing patterns during a session of deep meditative breathing you will be able to access and bring balance to both sides of your mind. This will have the effect of calming your mind and nervous system. Once again, by consciously controlling your breath you will be able to gain control and calm your body and mind. This is how you perform this relaxation technique.

1. While performing a session of diaphragmatic breathing use your right thumb to close off your right nostril.

2. Inhale slowly through your left nostril with a deep diaphragmatic breath for a count of 5.

3. Hold your breath for a count of 7.

4. Close your left nostril with your ring finger and release the thumb off your right nostril.

5. Exhale through your right nostril, completely emptying your lungs, for a count of 8.

6. Inhale slowly through your right nostril for a count of 5.

7. Hold your breath for a count of 7. As you do so release your left nostril and close your right with your thumb.

8. Breathe out through your left nostril for a count of 8.

This counts as one complete round of nasal breathing. I suggest you start slowly by performing one or two rounds at first and increasing that over time. Once again, if you have any kind of health issues such as high blood pressure, do not hold attempt to hold your breath. You may find at times that one of your nostrils is so congested that you cannot breathe out of it. Do not let this concern you. This simply means that you have caught your body at the height of it nostril-cleaning cycle. In these situations I suggest you simply wait for a bit until your nostril clears up enough to perform deep nasal breaths. Remember, deep breathing should always be a relaxing and calming experience. Not something you should force at any time.

CHAPTER 7: BREATHING EXERCISES FOR SPECIFIC CONDITIONS

The basic full diaphragmatic breath, along with the mudra and nasal breathing variations, are really all you need to improve your breathing. Simply practicing them in some form for 5 to 10 minutes a day will do wonders for your health and happiness. There are countless varieties of deep breathing exercises out there, however. What follows are a few I have come across that have helped others with various health conditions. You can either use them as a supplement to the basic diaphragmatic breath or perform them by themselves anytime throughout the day.

CHAPTER 8: DEEP BREATHING FOR INSOMNIA

Millions of people worldwide suffer from insomnia and poor sleep. To help alleviate this condition I would recommend you first have a cold shower right before you go to bed. I suggest you start with a mildly cold shower and gradually lower the temperature over the course of a five minute period. This has the effect of cooling your body and preparing it for sleep. Once you have finished with your cold shower, go lie down in a properly ventilated room and try performing one of these two deep breathing exercises:

Deep Breathing for Insomnia Variation #1

1. Begin by lying flat on your back in your bed with your hands by your sides, palms down.
2. Close your eyes. Begin to inhale through your nose as you simultaneously begin to raise your arms up over your head.
3. Continue to inhale, completely filling your lungs, until your arms are straight above your head on the ground. For every inhale you take your arms should move like this in a 180 degree fashion.

4. Hold this breath for a count of 8 to 10 seconds.

5. Begin to exhale slowly out of your nose as you raise your arms and return them to the starting

position. You should time it so that your arms come to rest beside you just as you finish exhaling.

6. Repeat this exercise 4 to 10 times or until you start to become drowsy. At this point you should be feeling very relaxed. You may find that listening to some gentle music may help loosen up as well.

Deep Breathing for Insomnia Variation #2

1. Get into bed and lie flat on your back.

2. Close your eyes and take a deep breath in through your nose as you slowly count to 5.

3. As you breathe in imagine you can see the air as it flows through your nose and into your lungs.

4. Hold this breath for a count of 4.

5. Exhale your lungs completely by breathing out through your nose for a count of 8.

6. Repeat this breathing technique 6 to 10 more times or until you start to feel drowsy.

Taking a cold shower before you perform this mediation and listening to some soothing music afterwards works well with this relaxation technique.

CHAPTER 9: ANTI-AGING BREATHING EXERCISES

As we age the breathing capacity of our lungs and the flexibility of our rib cage tends to diminish. These breathing exercises are designed to ameliorate these tendencies if not outright reverse them.

Anti-aging Breathing Exercise #1

This breathing exercise is meant to increase your lungs capacity to store air.

1. Begin by bending forward and placing the palms of your hands on your bent knees. Exhale all of the air from your lungs through your nose.

2. Begin to inhale through your nose as you slowly start to stand up straight.

3. As you continue to stand up straight, raise both of your arms over your head until your lungs are completely filled with air.

4. Hold your breath for a count of 8 seconds with your arms above your head.

5. Begin to exhale through your nose as you bend over at the waist and return to the starting position.

6. Repeat this movement 2 or 3 more times.

Anti-Aging Breathing Exercise #2

The aim of this breathing exercise is to help keep your rib cage flexible so that it can expand easily when you breathe.

1. Begin by standing with your arms by your sides. Exhale all of the air from your lungs through your nose.

2. Slowly inhale through your nose so that you completely fill your lungs.

3. Hold your breath while placing your palms on your hips with your pinkie fingers touching other on your back. Now pull your elbows back as far as you can while still holding your breath. Try to hold this position for a count of 10.

4. Slowly exhale through your nose as you lower your arms back by your sides.

5. Repeat this breathing exercise 2 or 3 more times.

CHAPTER 10: DEEP BREATHING EXERCISE FOR ASTHMA

Asthma is an all too common condition in which a person's airways become constricted, making breathing difficult. All the deep breathing exercises found in this book can help with this condition. What follows are some deep breathing exercises that some have found to be particularly effective.

Asthma Treatment #1 – Chest Expander

This breathing exercise will help you gain control over your inhalation and exhalation while expanding your chest. As you get stronger you can increase the amount of time you hold your breath. Just remember to only hold your breath to the point where you are comfortable. Never force yourself to hold your breath to the point where you feel faint or ill. Go slowly and listen to your body.

1. Begin with your arms straight out in front of you at shoulder level. Your palms should be facing each other.

2. Inhale through your nose for a count of 4 as you move your arms as far back as possible, which will help you expand your chest. As you do so imagine that you have a "life force" that exists between your palms. Sometimes I like to imagine this life force as a

ball of vibrant energy that has the potential to expel into the universe.

As you separate your palms, imagine this ball of energy growing and becoming more powerful. This visualization technique will help your mind focus to get the most out of your breathing and will really help energize you. The ball of energy you are seeing and feeling in your mind's eye is a representation of what you are actually doing in your lungs.

3. Hold your breath for a count of 4.

4. Exhale through your nose for a count of 4 as you bring your palms back together (shrinking the energy ball as you do so).

5. Perform this exercise for a minimum of 4 to 6 times or as long as you like.

Asthma Treatment #2 – Chest Extender

This breathing exercise is similar to asthma treatment #1 except we will be working on extending and expanding your chest forward. Once again as you get stronger you can work on holding your breath for longer periods of time.

1. Begin with your feet together and your palms facing each other near your chest.

2. As you inhale your breath through your nose for a count of 4 extend your arms forward away from your

chest. You should finish with your palms facing forward at shoulder level.

3. Hold your breath for another count of 4.

4. Exhale through your nose for a count of 4 as you bring your arms back to the starting position.

5. Repeat this breathing exercise 4 to 6 times.

Asthma Treatment #3

Candle Blowing - With this breathing exercise you will be purposely breathing out through your mouth instead of your nose for once. The reason for this is that it allows you to put gentle pressure on the lungs, which will work your diaphragm and other abdominal muscles.

1. Begin with your feet shoulder width apart and your hands on your hips just be- low your rib cage.

2. Inhale through your nose for a count of 4, completely filling your lungs.

3. Hold your breath for a count of 2.

4. Exhale slowly and steadily through your mouth. Purse your lips, almost like you're blowing out a candle. It should take you between 8 and 10 counts to completely exhale all of the air from your lungs.

5. Perform this exercise between 2 and 4 times.

CHAPTER 11: BREATHING EXERCISES FOR PANIC ATTACKS AND ANXIETY RELIEF

As I have already noted, your emotional state affects your breath. When you are experiencing anxiety, stress or panic your breath typically becomes shallow and quick. When you are aware of this, however, you can use your breath to reverse this process and gain control over your emotions. The next time you are experiencing a panic attack or some form of anxiety try the following:

1. First of all, use the thumb and forefinger of one hand to firmly massage the skin between the thumb and forefinger of the opposite hand. This is a form of self- acupressure that will help ease a nervous stomach. This technique by itself can also be helpful for motion sickness.

2. As you continue to massage your hands, concentrate on your breath. Breathe in deeply through your nose for a count of 4.

3. Hold your breath for a count of 4 as you roll your shoulders forwards and backwards a couple of times.

4. Exhale through your nose for a count of 4. Imagine you are blowing all of the stress and tension from your body as you do so.

5. After you've emptied your lungs, don't breathe in for a few seconds. Instead, force your stomach muscles in and out 4 times. 6. Breathe in again through your nose for a count of 4, and repeat this process 5 times. When you are done you should feel more relaxed and peaceful. Note that this exercise can be done either sitting or standing.

CHAPTER 12: A BREATHING EXERCISE FOR FATIGUE

Adenosine Triphosphate (or ATP for short) is a by-product of breathing that helps to regulate physical action and mood. During the day you may experience dips in your ATP levels, which can result in fatigue, aches and pain. This one breath meditation can help to reverse falling ATP levels and can be done anywhere at any time.

1. Sit in a comfortable chair with your back straight and your shoulders relaxed.

2. Close your eyes and inhale through your nose as slowly and deeply as you can. Imagine your body filling up with energizing oxygen from the bottom of your lungs to the top.

3. Hold your breath for a moment and then start to exhale through your nose as slowly as you can. Imagine you are releasing all of the tension and fatigue from your body. This one-minute refreshing breath can be done at home, during a workout, or any time you need a quick boost of energy. It will refresh and restore your body, mind and soul all at once. Give it a try and see for yourself.

CHAPTER 13: BREATHING EXERCISES FOR HAPPINESS

Aside from the myriad of other benefits already mentioned deep breathing can have the effect of instilling in the practitioner a sense of wellbeing and happiness. By itself deep diaphragmatic breathing can help lift feelings of depression and improve your mood. Although all deep-breathing exercises can have this effect, the following two methods we'll look at can accelerate the process. Please note though that when performing these exercises for the first time you may not be able to hold your breath for the full count at first. If you experience any discomfort at all, such as dizziness, return to the standing position immediately and relax until the feeling passes. As always go slowly and use common sense.

The Cleansing Breath

This breathing exercise will help to energize you while purging your body of negative emotions.

1. Begin by standing with your feet comfortably apart and your hands by your sides.

2. Inhale through your nose as you raise your arms above your head while bending your back backward. Bend as far back as you can comfortably while

looking at the sky until your lungs are completely filled with air.

3. Hold your breath in this position for 4 to 5 seconds.

4. Exhale through your nose as you bend forward at the waist. Keep your knees slightly bent as you do so. When you have bent forward as far as you can, make an effort to really suck your stomach in in order to expel every last bit of air possible.

5. Begin to inhale through your nose as you slowly start to stand up again, raising your hands above your head.

6. Repeat this motion 5 times.

THE HAPPINESS BREATH

The physical motion of the happiness breath is very similar to the cleansing breath. The difference between the two exercises is in how long and when you hold the breath. When done properly the happiness breath is excellent at recharging your brain while helping to clean out your skull cavities (such as your sinuses, ears and nose).

1. Just like the cleansing breath, begin by standing with your feet comfortably apart and your hands by your sides.

2. Inhale through your nose as you raise your arms above your head while bending your back backward. Bend as far back as you can comfortably while

looking at the sky until your lungs are completely filled with air.

3. Hold your breath as you bend forward at the waist. Keep your knees slightly bent as you do so. Bend forward as far as you can and attempt to continue to hold your breath for a count of 10.

4. Continue to hold your breath as you return to the standing position with your hands above your head.

5. Bend forward again as you now exhale all of the breath through your nose.

6. Inhale through your nose as you slowly start to stand up again, raising your hands above your head.

7. Repeat this motion 5 times.

CHAPTER 14: BREATHING EXERCISES FOR HEALTHY LIVING AND ENERGY

Reach for the Sky

1. Begin by standing with your feet comfortably together and your hands on your shoulders.

2. As you begin to inhale through your nose start to raise your hands upwards with the palms down. You should time the inhale with the raising motion of your hands so that your lungs are completely filled with oxygen when your arms are fully extended.

3. Exhale through your nose as you lower your hands back to your shoulders. Your lungs should be completely empty by the time your hands touch your shoulders.

4. Repeat this motion 10 times.

Hands Forward

1. Begin by standing with your feet comfortably together and your hands on your shoulders. This is the starting position.

2. As you begin to inhale through your nose extend your hands straight out in front of you with your palms facing forward. Your lungs should be completely filled

with oxygen by the time your arms reach the point of maximum extension.

3. Exhale through your nose as you return your hands to the starting position. Your lungs should be completely empty by the time your hands reach your shoulders.

4. Repeat this motion 10 times.

Hands to the Side

1. Begin by standing with your feet comfortably together and your hands on your shoulders. This is the starting position.

2. As you begin to inhale through your nose extend your hands to either side with your palms facing outward. Your lungs should be completely filled with oxygen when your arms reach the point of maximum extension.

3. Exhale through your nose as you return your hands to the starting position. Your lungs should be completely empty by the time your hands reach your shoulders.

4. Repeat this motion 10 times.

CONCLUSION

In our modern world, we tend get so caught up in "daily life" that we neglect paying attention to our body. By practicing the methods mentioned in this book, you will hopefully be able to create a more healthy, happy, and satisfying life.

PREVENTING CANCER THE NATURAL WAY

PREVENT. OVERCOME. EMBRACE

Cancer: Beginner's Guide to Preventing Cancer the Natural Way

I.   Introduction to Cancer (statistics, causes, treatment, prognosis)

II.   Risk Factors

III. Natural methods of cancer prevention

    a. Diet and Nutrition

    b. Top foods with cancer-fighting properties

    c. Top alkaline foods

    d. Supplements / Superfoods

    e. Exercise

    f. Sleep

    g. Environmental toxins

IV.   Conclusion

The cancer industry is easily the most lucrative industry in the world today. Thousands of businesses are successfully making a profit from the current $125 billion in medical costs for cancer patients alone. However, various research conducted around the world prove that there are alternative ways of preventing cancer using natural means. Yet the cancer industry, which employs millions and earns even more, continues to prosper while trying to hide the fact that cancer can be prevented.

Simply put, the cancer industry is so lucrative, that incentive to "discover" a cure could potentially affect many of those who are reaping in the rewards. But natural cures and preventive measures are all around us; all one needs to do is look for the information which is widely available.

In this book, we will explore cancer – discuss what it's about, who's at risk, and how you can prevent it without having to spend your life savings or potentially go into debt.

I.   Introduction to Cancer

Cancer is the collective term given to a broad range of diseases where the body's cells divide uncontrollably. Normal cells can divide in an orderly method: when these cells are damaged or old, new cells grow to take their place. On the other hand, cancer cells tend to crowd normal cells, making it difficult for the body to function the way it should. When cells become abnormal, the damaged or old cells that should have died survive, while new cells grow even if they are not needed. When these extra cells continue to divide, they may form a growth called a tumor. Many kinds of cancers result in a solid tumor or a mass of tissue, although others, such as leukemia or cancer of the blood, do not.

The human body contains trillions of cells, and cancer can begin anywhere: lungs, colon, blood, or even the bone. Many cancers are similar to each other although they differ in how their cells grow, and how they spread around the body.

There are two kinds of tumors: malignant and benign. Malignant refers to tumors that are cancerous and thus can invade surrounding tissues. When tumors grow, some cancer cells can travel around the body through the lymph system or blood, and form a new tumor elsewhere. Benign tumors do not spread into nearby tissues, although they can sometimes grow into large sizes. Benign tumors may be removed

through surgery and oftentimes do not grow back although in some instances malignant tumors do. Most benign tumors are not fatal unless it is located in the brain.

Symptoms of Cancer

Because cancer refers to a wide range of diseases, the signs and symptoms vary greatly depending on the location of the cancer, its size, how much it has affected the tissue or organ, and if it has metastasized (spread). When cancer grows, it can cause added pressure or pain to nearby nerves, organs, or blood vessels. If the cancer is a critical location such as the brain, small tumors can already cause symptoms. Some forms of cancer are easier to identify, such as breast or skin cancer, because they form distinguishable lumps outside or underneath the skin.

Some cancers don't show signs or symptoms until they are already quite large. Certain cancers may result in weight loss, fatigue, or fever because the excess cells use the body's energy reserves or release substances that affect how the body converts energy from food. Cancer may also cause the immune system to produce these symptoms.

The general signs of cancer may be difficult to detect because more often than not they do not mean that one has cancer. However, if these symptoms are persistent and do not go away, it's best to see a doctor:

- Fever
- Fatigue

- Unexplained weight loss
- Changes in skin color
- Pain

Treatment

Cancer treatment is always more effective in cases where it is identified early especially when it is smaller and hasn't yet metastasized.

Doctors can perform surgery to remove the cancer as well as other body parts that are affected by the cancer. It is common to remove part or the entire breast in cases of breast cancer. Prostate glands may be removed for prostate cancer.

Chemotherapy utilizes drugs to kill cancer cells and preventing them from dividing. Chemotherapy drugs are powerful and can affect many other growing and healthy cells. This may result in side effects such as fatigue, muscle pain, headaches, stomach pain, pain caused by nerve damage, oral sores, nausea, diarrhea, vomiting, changes in cognitive ability, fertility issues, blood disorders, hair loss, and appetite loss to name a few.

Radiation therapy uses high-energy x-rays to destroy and slow down the growth of cancer cells. It may be used either alone or in conjunction with chemotherapy or surgery. Radiation may result in side effects such as fatigue, skin problems, and the possibility of developing cancer again later on. In addition, the side effects borne from radiation tend to be localized depending on the area that radiation therapy is targeting.

Prognosis

The prognosis for cancer depends on several factors:

- Type of cancer
- Location of cancer in the body
- Stage of cancer
- If the cancer has spread
- Patient's age and status of health prior to cancer
- How the patient responds to treatment
- The cancer's grade

II.   Risk Factors

It can be difficult to explain why one person gets cancer and another doesn't. However, research shows that risk factors can increase the chances that a person may develop cancer at some point in their life. Cancer risk factors include behaviors as well as exposure to substances or chemicals, which are controllable. However, certain cancer risk factors, such as family history and age, cannot be controlled.

In this chapter, we will explore the most widely studied suspected risk factors for cancer. Avoiding exposure to controllable risk factors can lower your risk of developing some cancers.

1. **Age**:

    The average age for cancer diagnosis is 66 years old; thus older age increases one's proclivity to developing cancer although it can occur at any age. Certain kinds of cancers such as neuroblastoma are more prevalent in children rather than adults.

2. **Alcohol use**:

    Alcohol consumption can increase risk for throat, mouth, liver, larynx, and breast cancer. When alcohol is combined with tobacco use, cancer risk skyrockets. However with certain cancer-fighting properties such as resveratrol present in red wine, recommended consumption is up to 2 glasses daily.

3. **Hormones**:

    Although hormones play an important role in men and women, estrogen has been associated with an increase in cancer risk. Women who take combined menopausal hormone therapy which contains estrogen plus progestin can increase the risk of breast cancer. Research shows that breast cancer risk is linked to the progesterone and estrogen produced by the ovaries. Prolonged exposure to these hormones, such as when a woman starts menstruation at an early age, never giving birth, going through a late menopause, or when the first pregnancy is at a later age, all increases a woman's risk of acquiring breast cancer.

4. **Obesity**:

   Overweight people are at risk for several cancers while staying at a healthy weight and maintaining an active lifestyle reduces the risk of cancer.

5. **Radiation**:

   Exposure to ionizing radiation found in x-rays, radon, gamma rays and other sources of high energy radiation can damage DNA and result in cancer. Non-ionizing forms of radiation such as those found in cellphones as well as magnetic fields are not intense enough to cause DNA damage or cancer.
   a. Radon is a form of radioactive gas found in soil and rocks. People living in areas that contain high levels of radon in its

soil and rocks are more vulnerable to developing lung cancer later on.

b. High energy radiation sources include medical procedures that utilize x-rays, positron emission tomography (PET) scan, and computed tomography (CT) scans; alpha particles, beta particles, gamma rays, and neutrons are strong enough to result in DNA damage as well as cancer. Aside from hospital procedures, high energy radiation can also be released as a result of accidents in nuclear power plants.

6. **Sunlight**:

Exposure to the sun and tanning booths gives off ultraviolet (UV) rays which can cause skin damage and skin cancer. The amount of time spent under the sun and in tanning beds should be limited by people of all ages to reduce risk of developing skin cancer. In addition, UV radiation can also be reflected by water, ice, sand, and snow; thus, anyone exposed should use proper protection by means of protective clothing and sunscreen with at least a sun protection factor of 15. Other useful ways of limiting UV radiation outdoors is by wearing long-sleeved clothing, sunglasses, and wide-brimmed hats.

7. Tobacco:

Tobacco use and cigarette smoking is the number one cause of cancer worldwide. People who are often around others who smoke cigarettes are also at risk of developing cancer due to exposure to second-hand smoke because the smoke emitted by cigarettes contains enough chemicals to cause damage to DNA. Tobacco use can result in several cancers including larynx, lung, esophagus, mouth, bladder, liver, kidney and many more. Those who use smokeless tobacco are also at risk of developing cancers of the mouth, pancreas, and throat. When it comes to tobacco use, zero tolerance is recommended for anyone who wants to reduce their cancer risk because there is no such thing as a safe amount of tobacco to smoke.

III.   Preventing Cancer Through Natural Means

Despite what the cancer industry says, it is possible to prevent cancer naturally. The key to preventing cancer is in your lifestyle: the food you eat, the amount of exercise you get, the chemicals and toxins your body is exposed to, and your sleeping habits all play a role. The good news is that all of these factors can be controlled. It is also important to remember that while there is no one food that will prevent cancer altogether, successful prevention lies in the combination of efforts that are described here later on.

Cancer doesn't develop overnight but by making these changes to your lifestyle, you can significantly reduce your risk of developing it later on.

a. Diet and Nutrition

Food contains a variety of components that aid in cancer prevention: these include vitamins, minerals, macronutrients, and phytonutrients from plants. The National Cancer Institute states that as much as 80% of cancers are due to specific lifestyle factors; 30% of these are due to smoking and as much as 50% are associated with a poor diet. What you eat and what you don't eat can have a significant effect on your overall health. Certain foods can increase your risk of cancer; similarly, you may be neglecting important foods that can dramatically reduce your risk.

In addition, research has also been conducted that emphasizes there is a link between an acidic body and cancer risk. Cancer, as well as many other preventable diseases such as diabetes and arthritis, can only grow in an acidic environment and also cannot survive in an alkaline environment. Those who develop cancer have acidic bodies and low pH levels. Certain foods can either increase the acidity in one's body and thus an ideal diet for cancer prevention is one that raises the body's alkalinity.

What To Avoid

- Genetically modified organisms (GMO's) and pesticides:

  GMO's may be plants or animals whose DNA has been manipulated to be resistant to pesticides. Studies have shown that farmers who are exposed to genetically modified crops and pesticides have a higher incidence of developing cancer. Consumption of genetically modified animals or crops can also increase one's risk of developing certain cancers such as brain tumors, breast cancer, and leukemia among others.

- Processed meat:

Processed meat refers to any meat that has been altered to change its taste or extend its shelf life. The most common methods used in processed meat include curing, smoking, or adding preservatives. Popular forms of processed meat include corned beef, hotdogs, sausages, bacon, ham, canned meat, beef jerky, and meat-based sauces. Not only is meat an acid-forming food, but the chemicals used in processing these meats are highly carcinogenic. Cooking in high temperatures such as barbecue or grilling also creates carcinogenic chemicals. While no red meat is best, medium or rare is a better choice. Any food that is charred, even toast, should be avoided.

- Farmed fish:

Dioxins, toxaphene, PCB's, and dieldrin- all cancer-causing substances have been found in high concentrations in farmed salmon which is present on most grocery store shelves and served in restaurants. Other varieties of farm-bred fish, including tilapia, contain high amounts of pesticides and antibiotics that are used to keep them alive.

- <u>Refined sugar:</u>

Commonly known as sucrose, refined sugar is derived from sugar beet or sugar cane. Sucrose is present in white and brown sugar that is used to make cakes, cookies, and to sweeten coffee. Refined sugar is also found in high-fructose corn syrup which is present in flavored yogurt, salad dressings, and tomato sauce. These sugars are linked to obesity-related cancers and its consumption also increases the body's acidity levels.

- <u>Canned food:</u>

Cans contain a carcinogen bisphenol-A (BPA) which has been linked to breast and prostate cancer incidence. It is a synthetic estrogen that can disrupt hormones even with minimal exposure. Canned tomatoes contain the highest levels of BPA because its high acidity causes BPA to leech from the cans. BPA is also present in a number of household products including utensils, microwave ovenware, and some baby bottles.

- <u>Aspartame:</u>

Commonly found in artificial sweeteners such as NutraSweet and Equal, aspartame has been linked to several illnesses as well as cancer. Research has shown that the chemicals contained in aspartame and other artificial sweeteners produce a deadly toxin in the body called DKP which in turn can produce carcinogens when it is being processed in the body.

<u>"Diet" and "Low-fat" food:</u>

Any frozen or pre-packaged food that is labeled "diet" or "low-fat" either contain aspartame, refined ingredients, high levels of sodium, and artificial flavoring to give it taste.

- <u>Excess salt:</u>

While salt consumption is necessary for health, too much salt can result in cancer and many other illnesses. The recommended dosage for salt should be under 1,500 milligrams of sodium per day.

- <u>Junk food:</u>

The consumption of junk food puts you at risk for cancer, obesity, and a host of other diseases:

  - Soft drinks and soda: The caramel food coloring that is widely used to give the beverage its brownish hue produces 4-MEI, which is a carcinogen. In addition, soft drinks contain high amounts of sugar in various forms; the consumption of sugar alters the body's pH in the intestines and increase acidity.

- Snacks that contain trans-fat: The most common snacks containing trans-fat include French fries, potato chips, deep fried foods, margarine, frosting, shortening, microwaved popcorn, chips (tortilla, potato, corn), and creamer.

What to Eat

- Fruits and vegetables:

Consuming fresh produce in all colors is an ideal way to ensure that you are getting maximum protection from cancer. Fruits and vegetables are rich in antioxidants including vitamins C and E, beta-carotene, and selenium which protect the body from cancer and aid in efficient functioning of organs and tissues.

As a general rule of thumb, fruits and vegetables have more potent cancer-fighting properties when they are altered as little as possible from the way they came out of the ground. This means that the less they are peeled or cooked, the better. Going organic is a better option especially if you intend to consume the skin of a fruit or vegetable as it is the skin exposed to pesticides. Also, while there is no need to go completely vegetarian in order to prevent cancer, you can achieve a balance by ensuring you add whole fruits and vegetables to each meal.

- Whole grains:

  Whole grains are important sources of fiber, protein, and magnesium. There are several kinds of whole grains to choose from, all of which are hearty, filling and flavorful. These include whole-wheat bread, corn, brown rice, barley, oatmeal, faro, millet, and others. Whole grains are more nutritious because they contain cancer-fighting phytochemicals while helping keep the digestive system functioning optimally. Other healthy compounds that are found in whole grains include saponins, lignans, flavonoids, phytic acid, and protease inhibitors.

- Legumes:

  Split peas, dry beans, and lentils are not only an excellent source of fiber and protein, but they are also rich in cancer-fighting compounds that include: lignans, saponins, resistant starch, and several phytochemicals.

- Coffee:

  A cup of good quality coffee may be an important source of antioxidant phytochemicals and riboflavin. However, the amount of antioxidants in coffee depends largely on how the coffee is prepared as well as how the beans are grown.

b. Top Foods with Cancer-Fighting Properties

Adding these foods to your daily diet will help boost immunity and provide you with nutrients and vitamins all while reducing your risk of cancer.

1. **Berries**

   are rich in potent antioxidants that fight cell-damaging free radicals. Berries also contain natural components that prevent cancer from spreading or growing.

2. **Tomatoes**

   are rich in lycopene, an antioxidant that may reduce the risk for certain cancers including breast and prostate.

3. **Green tea**

contains catechins which are associated with a lower risk of cancer. Sipping a cup or two of green tea a day also prevents free radicals from causing cell damage.

4. **Turmeric**

is an orange colored spice which is widely used in Indian cuisine. It contains curcumin which helps inhibit the growth of cancer cells and protects the liver from cirrhosis. Turmeric may be taken in capsule form or added as a powder into curries and other dishes.

5. **Grapes**

contain an antioxidant known as resveratrol which may be beneficial in inhibiting cancer growth. Resveratrol is found in grape juice as well as red wine and has been shown to lower risk of prostate cancer.

6. **Dark chocolate**

that contains at least 70% cocoa or cacao is rich in therapeutic polyphenols and antioxidants that help fight cancer. Catechins, in particular, are also present in dark chocolates.

7. **Nuts and seeds**

   can help reduce risk of developing certain
   cancers, particularly those found in the list
   below:

8. **Healthiest nuts**

   Walnuts
   Almonds
   Pecans
   Brazil nuts
   Cedar nuts

9. **Healthiest seeds**

   Hemp
   Sunflower
   Sesame
   Pumpkin
   Chia

c. Top Alkaline Foods

These foods can be integrated into your daily diet
to help your body attain an alkaline state:

1. **Cruciferous vegetables**

are easy to prepare in nutritious recipes while others can be tossed into a blender to supercharge your smoothie. These include:

- Arugula
- Basil
- Beet greens
- Bokchoy
- Broccoli
- Brussel sprouts
- Cabbage
- Celery
- Chard
- Spinach
- Kale

2. **Root vegetables**

can be eaten raw, steamed, roasted, or sautéed. These include:

- Beets
- Carrots
- Garlic
- Ginger
- Kohlrabi
- Onion
- Parsnips

- Sweet potato
- Turnips
- Yuca root

3. **Leafy greens**

are not only alkaline vegetables but are also packed with vitamins and nutrients. Their alkalizing qualities are more beneficial when eaten raw but light consuming them lightly steamed or marinated will also do. An effective and delicious way of consuming leafy greens is also by adding them to juices or smoothies.

- Cabbage
- Collard greens
- Dandelion greens
- Kale
- Mustard greens
- Romaine lettuce
- Turnip greens
- Spinach
- Swiss chard
- Watercress

4. **Lemons**

are recognized as a highly alkaline food which is also extremely versatile. Drinking lemon water daily is an easy way to maximize the alkalizing effects of lemon on the body. Lemon juice can be used to season many dishes and salads.

5. Cucumbers

make a great base for soups and can easily be added to juices and smoothies. They are one of the most alkaline vegetables and are also rich in vitamins A and C, manganese, potassium, magnesium, and folate. Cucumbers are water-rich and make filling snacks for any time of the day. Cucumber and lemon slices in water will also give you a delicious-tasting alkaline water.

d. Supplements and Superfoods

These superfoods and vitamins are a great addition to your diet. They are extremely nutritious and possess powerful cancer-fighting properties. Before taking any of these supplements or superfoods, it is best to talk to your doctor first.

- **Spirulina**,

  a blue-green algae, thrives in alkaline warm-water lakes. Spirulina derives its color from the protein phycocyanin, which can slow down the growth of cancer cells. Just like other plants and algae, spirulina is also rich in chlorophyll which has the ability to bind with cancer cells and promote its excretion from the body before they group into colonies and form tumors within the body. Spirulina may be taken in capsule or powder form.

- **Cacao**

  nibs contain high amounts of flavonoids which may prevent cancer and other illnesses including Alzheimer's. Flavonoids help prevent cellular damage caused by free radicals. In addition, cacao nibs are also rich in fiber, another key nutrient that helps in cancer prevention. Cacao nibs are best enjoyed raw, added to shakes, yogurts, and breakfast bowls.

- **Moringa,**

  a plant that grows in tropical areas of the world, is highly prized for its medicinal properties. Moringa is a powerful source of vitamin c, vitamin a, iron, calcium, potassium, and protein. In India, moringa plant is cultivated for its anti-tumor, anti-inflammatory, and anti-cancer properties. The plant contains a total of 36 anti-inflammatory agents, making it one of the most potent anti-cancer plants in the world. Moringa may be consumed in capsule, tablet, or powder form.

- **Chlorella**

  is freshwater seaweed or green algae that are recognized for its cancer-fighting properties. It is an excellent source of chlorophyll, protein, B vitamins, carbohydrates, amino acids, vitamin c, and vitamin e. Chlorella's nutritional content makes it a powerful defense in keeping the immune system strong enough to stave off inflammation and cancer. It is also taken by cancer patients to help their bodies tolerate chemotherapy more effectively. Chlorella is widely used in Japan where its healing qualities are well-known. Chlorella may be taken in capsule, tablet, or powder form.

- **Virgin coconut oil**

  derived from coconut trees is rich in immune-boosting and cancer-fighting properties. Its potent antioxidant properties have the ability to reverse cellular damage that may result in cancer while providing protection from free radicals. Virgin coconut oil is also rich in lauric acid which helps to kill viruses, bacteria, yeast, and parasites. It is also one of the most versatile oils in the world, providing people with health benefits regardless of which way it is used. Coconut oil is widely used as a cooking oil; it can be heated several times over without producing free radicals thus cooking with coconut oil can reduce cancer risk. Raw, virgin, organic coconut oil is ideal for cancer prevention; it is best taken in raw form orally. It can also be taken in capsule form or added directly to food.

Supplements

- **Coenzyme Q10**

  may reduce cancer risk while large
  amounts can inhibit breast cancer growth
  while boosting immunity. Recommended
  dosage of CoQ10 for cancer prevention is
  100mg per day.

- **Lycopene**

  supplements help prevent cellular damage
  caused by free radicals. Research has also
  shown that taking lycopene supplements
  may be able to reduce prostate tumors and
  inhibit growth. Recommended dosage for
  prostate cancer prevention is 10mg daily
  even if your diet already contains lycopene-
  rich foods.

- **Selenium**

  contains an antioxidant enzyme that helps
  the liver detoxify cancer-causing toxins.
  Studies show that 200 micrograms of

selenium taken daily can significantly reduce one's risk of developing lung, colon, and prostate cancers.

- **Vitamin K**

  can reduce the risk for cancers of the liver and the breast. The recommended dosage is 300 micrograms of vitamin K-1 or K-2.

e. Exercise

Regular exercise can significantly reduce the risk of getting several cancers, including breast, bowel, prostate, and womb. Ideally, 30 minutes of rigorous exercise or an hour of moderate activity is recommended.

Physical activity can combat cancer by fighting inflammation and reducing obesity. Inflammation is the immune system's response to injury which is often caused by pathogens. Common characteristics of inflammation include increased blood flow, redness, swelling, and pain. These can occur in wounds outside the body as well as in organs and tissues that are not immediately visible to the human eye. Chronic inflammation can happen even if there is no injury because it results in DNA damage. Studies have shown that humans who experience inflammation for long periods of time are at higher risk of developing cancer. For example, those who suffer from chronic inflammatory bowel diseases such as Crohn disease are at higher risk for colon cancer. A physically active body produces more antioxidants which are necessary for fighting the free radicals that cause inflammation.

Exercise is also an effective way to deal with stress, which triggers inflammation. Chronic stress can alter immune cells even before they enter the bloodstream, making them ready to fight infection even when there is no injury which then leads to inflammation.

Furthermore, regular exercise is crucial for keeping excess weight off. Obesity is linked to several cancers including breast, esophagus, pancreas, colon, gallbladder, kidney, and endometrium. There are several facts that link obesity with cancer:

- The blood of obese people have been shown to contain higher levels of insulin growth factor 1 (IGF-1) and insulin which has been shown to increase risk for certain cancers.
- Adipose tissue produces excess estrogen, an occurrence that has been tied to endometrial, breast, and other kinds of cancers.
- Obesity leads to chronic sub-level inflammation, which thus increases one's cancer risk.

f. Sleep

Adequate sleep is crucial for disease prevention and ensuring your body is performing at its optimal best. Prolonged periods of impaired sleep have been linked to cancer and quicker growth of tumors. Studies show that men who have difficulties sleeping well had higher incidence of prostate cancer, and inadequate sleep may result in the recurrence of breast cancer while increasing the risk of developing more aggressive forms of breast cancer in women.

Less than 6 hours of sleep a night can increase the risk for colorectal adenoma which can result in cancer. In general, people who sleep less than 6 hours at night increased cancer risk by as much as 50% when compared to those who got at least 7 hours of sleep a night.

Insulin resistance combined with disrupted melatonin production is two primary processes which can increase cancer risk as a result of poor sleep. Furthermore, insufficient sleep decreases the levels of leptin in the body which are necessary for regulating fat resulting in increased levels of ghrelin, a hunger hormone.

Therefore, those who don't get adequate sleep are more prone to overeating and gaining excess weight. Overweight women are most affected by the insulin resistance and weight gain risk factors. Breast cancer is the most prevalent form of cancer in women, yet women who are obese are as much as 60% more prone due to the insulin resistance that occurs as a result of poor sleep habits. Breast cancers are fueled by the body's estrogen production which increases when a woman has more fat.

In addition, those who work the night shift are at higher risk of developing cancer and a host of other illnesses. Hormone disruptions are likely the primary cause of cancer in those who work night shifts. Even if you live a healthy lifestyle and eat the right foods, getting inadequate sleep can discount all of these and still put you at risk for cancer.

g. Environmental toxins

1. Household cleaners

People oftentimes don't realize how many chemicals they are allowing themselves to be exposed to simply by using household cleaners. Switching to natural and environmentally safe household products is an easy and inexpensive way to make your home cancer-free. It's also relatively easy and inexpensive to make your own natural household cleaners using lemons, vodka, soap, or vinegar mixed diluted in water.

Several of the chemicals found in common household cleaners can cause cancer and thus any product containing these should be avoided:

- Synthetic musks
- Terpenes
- Phenol
- Phthalates
- Benzene
- Petroleum solvents
- Butyl cellosolve
- Nonylphenol ethoxylates (NPE)
- Styrene
- 1,4-diclorobenzene
- Formaldehyde
- Triclosan

Beauty Products

Personal care products may seem beneficial to use at first, but once you start examining product labels you may be surprised to find cancer-causing chemicals lurking in your shampoo or body lotion. Skin exposure to these chemicals increases is even worse than ingesting them because the skin absorbs them immediately and it goes directly into the bloodstream.

The most common chemicals found in personal and beauty care products to avoid include:

- Sodium lauryl sulfate (SLS)
- Paraben
- Musks
- 1,4 –Dioxane
- Phthalates
- Antibacterials
- Mineral oil
- Paraffin
- Petroleum
- Hydroquinone
- Mercury
- Lead
- Formaldehyde
- Nano particles

A good rule of thumb when it comes to personal care products is if you wouldn't eat it then it probably isn't safe enough to use on your skin. Use organic, all-natural, and vegan products on your face and body whenever possible.

IV.   Conclusion

Cancer is a disease dreaded by people worldwide, understandably so as it causes millions of deaths every year. The cancer industry adds to the stigma, given the fact that the business is considered lucrative. Too little is done to educate people on how cancer can be prevented naturally and thus many people end up feeling helpless when it comes to understanding what changes can be made in order to reduce one's risk for cancer. Keep in mind that more than half of all cancer deaths could have easily been prevented by taking simple steps such as quitting cigarettes, eating the proper food, getting enough exercise, and living a healthy lifestyle. These things are not rocket-science – but by taking the first step forward in understanding what you can change today, you are well on your way to a cancer-free life.

www.ingramcontent.com/pod-product-compliance
Lightning Source LLC
Chambersburg PA
CBHW062105280526
45788CB00003B/1354